Contents

About the Author

Epigraph

"The path to sovereignty lies not in dominance over others, but in the mastery of oneself and the harmony of all things."

Unknown Sage

"What lies behind us and what lies before us are tiny matters compared to what lies within us."

Ralph Waldo Emerson

Dedication & Acknowledgment

This journey would not have been possible without many's guidance, inspiration, and support.

To my family, whose encouragement and belief in my vision never wavered – thank you for being my sanctuary.

To the countless readers and dreamers who find solace and strength in stories, your voices and dreams breathe life into this work.

A special thanks to the mentors who have shared their wisdom and reminded me of the importance of staying rooted yet reaching for the stars.

And to the natural world, whose beauty and resilience continue to inspire – thank you for being the silent teacher of harmony and sovereignty.

To those who dare to seek their truth and to the quiet places where wisdom whispers to those who listen. May you find your path and walk it with courage and grace.

Foreword

We live in a time when searching for meaning, and self-realization feels more urgent than ever.

In a world brimming with distractions and challenges, the concept of sovereignty – not as dominion over others.

But as the profound alignment of one's inner and outer worlds – resonates deeply.

Jack's journey is a mirror to our own lives. It challenges us to reflect on our purpose, reconnect with the world, and embrace our power to create harmony within and around us. It is not merely a tale of adventure and transformation; It is an invitation to embark on your journey of self-discovery.

As you delve into the chapters ahead, may Jack's experiences inspire and empower you.

May his triumphs remind you of your strength, and his lessons illuminate your path.

Together, let us step forward into a world of possibility, with courage in our hearts and sovereignty in our souls.

With gratitude and hope,

Sabrina Winterstone

Introduction

In a world teetering on the edge of chaos, one man's odyssey into the heart of self-discovery and sovereignty inspires us all to awaken the dormant power within.

Jack is an inquisitive and independent teenager from a small town in Australia. His parents are both educators who encouraged critical thinking and self-reliance from a young age. Growing up, Jack often felt out of place among his peers, drawn more to deep questions about life, freedom, and purpose than to the typical teenage pursuits.

Jack has recently finished high school and is taking a gap year before starting university. Instead of following the traditional path, he decides to embark on a journey through Europe to uncover what it means to live a sovereign life – one that is free, purposeful, and aligned with his values.

"Jack's Journey to Sovereignty" is a tale of courage, destiny, and transformation, set against a backdrop of mystical realms and ancient wisdom.

Through Jack's quest, readers can reflect on their lives and uncover the harmony and resilience needed to navigate an ever-changing world.

Join Jack as he charts a path toward enlightenment, weaving together timeless truths and profound lessons that echo across generations.

CHAPTER ONE

The Awakening

JACK'S PEACEFUL VILLAGE EXISTENCE shifts when he discovers a secret grove in the forest. Enchanted by an ancient tree, its murmurs of authority awaken a fire in him. The village elders, noticing Jack's bond with the tree's knowledge, urge him to delve into its deeper insights.

Jack's journey starts with the understanding that sovereignty is discovered rather than given. While he listens to the tree, he recognizes the interconnectedness of all life. This insight transforms his view, marking the initial steps of his adventure.

The sacred grove transforms into Jack's sanctuary, a place where he feels a deep connection to the universe. The dappled sunlight that filters through the ancient branches appears to convey messages only he can understand. Meditating under the tree, Jack absorbs its lessons and finds comfort in its timeless presence. The twisted, deep roots seem to anchor him to a profound and unchanging truth.

Jack's extraordinary bond with nature starts to motivate others in the village. Both friends and strangers turn to him for guidance, captivated by the changes they observe in him. They remark on his serene demeanor, emerging wisdom, and talent for appreciating beauty in everyday life. Jack's evolution turns into a symbol of hope.

The village elders show great interest in Jack, sharing their wisdom and stories. These interactions bolster Jack's determination to follow his path. They talk about the importance of balancing action with reflection, encouraging him to integrate both as he progresses.

In moments of solitude and reflection, Jack senses the burden of responsibility. He realizes that his journey extends beyond his needs to those seeking hope from him. He acknowledges that his decisions will have far-reaching effects, influencing the lives of others in ways he has yet to comprehend and foresee.

The ancient tree's whispers become more distinct, guiding Jack on his journey. Each message acts like a puzzle piece, slowly revealing the bigger picture of his destiny. The tree's voice, sometimes gentle and at other times commanding, sparks a pressing urge in him to venture further beyond known.

The village undergoes a gentle transformation as its residents grow more aware and harmonious. Jack's evolution creates a ripple effect, inspiring others in the community. Simple gestures of kindness increase and the previously unappreciated beauty of their environment is gradually recognized and cherished.

Before leaving the village, Jack enjoys a last evening in the grove. He expresses gratitude to the tree for its wisdom, vowing to return with tales from his travels. Beneath the starry sky, he senses both an ending and a new beginning, as if the universe is encouraging him to move forward.

Filled with both excitement and anxiety, Jack departs the village, entering a realm of opportunities and obstacles. Though the path forward is unclear, he holds a strong sense of purpose within.

CHAPTER TWO

Beyond the Village

STEPPING AWAY FROM THE comfort of home, Jack embarks on an adventure into unfamiliar territory. Every new environment introduces him to people searching for meaning. Through his exchanges, he uncovers the commonality of his journey and the collective human desire for purpose harmony.

Through trials and encounters, Jack's confidence grows. He learns that sovereignty requires resilience and an open heart. The seeds of wisdom from the ancient tree begin to blossom as Jack inspires others to embrace their unique paths.

Jack's first stop is a bustling town where he meets a merchant struggling with self-doubt. The merchant's livelihood is failing, and his days are consumed by fear and hesitation.

Jack engages the merchant in conversation, guiding him to rediscover his original passion for his craft. Their dialogue creates a profound effect, with the merchant's revitalized spirit igniting transformation in his work community.

The challenges of travel challenge Jack's patience and determination. Severe weather and strange landscapes compel him to draw on his acquired lessons. Nights under the stars instill humility and thankfulness in him; the immensity of the world highlights his modest but meaningful existence place.

In a secluded village, Jack meets a healer who recounts her path of self-discovery. Their shared wisdom marks a pivotal moment in Jack's grasp of interconnectedness. The healer's stories of resilience and her profound bond with nature motivate Jack to enhance his understanding practices.

Jack starts maintaining a journal to record his thoughts and experiences. This habit evolves into a source of solace and introspection throughout his journey. Through writing, he navigates his experiences and identifies patterns in his personal development, transforming his travels into a rich tapestry of connections lessons.

One evening, Jack discovers a circle of travelers gathered around a campfire. Their animated stories and laughter evoke in him the significance of community. These brief instances of connection serve as anchors, reassuring Jack that he is never alone on his journey path.

Jack's reputation begins to rise. He becomes known as a seeker of sovereignty, bringing hope to those around him. News spreads about the young man who listens intently and speaks with wisdom beyond his years years.

As Jack explores further, he realizes that the world is expansive and intimate. Although cultures vary, he uncovers universal human connections that bind us all. Each encounter reveals to him that sovereignty is not an isolated endeavor but rather a collective journey of development and understanding.

A serendipitous meeting with a traveling musician reveals to Jack the significance of art and self-expression. The musician's melodies, rich with tales of yearning and happiness, strike a profound chord within him, enhancing Jack's personal journey. He understands that true sovereignty involves not only learning but also crafting one's narrative, leading him to integrate creativity into his life's path.

Chapter Three

Trials of the Heart

JACK'S JOURNEY PRESENTS HIM with significant challenges that test his resilience and his beliefs' strength. As he dives deeper into the unknown, he encounters experiences that challenge the core of his spirit, compelling him to face his vulnerabilities and fears.

Jack's initial significant challenge is betrayal. A reliable friend whom he aided earlier betrays him for selfish reasons. The pain of this betrayal forces Jack to re-evaluate his judgment and his compassion for others. After days of contemplation, he comes to understand that sovereignty involves recognizing that he cannot always control others' actions; he can only control how he responds to them.

During his darkest moments, Jack learns the importance of forgiveness for himself and others. He recalls the teachings from the ancient tree, understanding that growth frequently arises from discomfort and hardship. This insight brings him peace amidst the chaos and guides him toward a journey of inner healing.

Jack finds peace in a tranquil forest in one of his lowest moments. The gentle sounds of nature calm his restless mind. Watching a stream effortlessly navigate around barriers, he derives a profound metaphor for his life: being flexible and adaptable amid challenges and adversity.

An unexpected encounter with a wise elder provides Jack with the guidance he seeks. The elder, who has journeyed through various experiences, recounts her tale of loss and healing, highlighting the significance of remaining faithful to one's inner compass. Her insights rejuvenate Jack's resolve and remind him of his aspiration's purpose.

Jack's journey through struggles is not alone. He encounters others facing challenges, too. Together, they create a temporary yet profoundly connected community. By sharing their hardships and triumphs, they strengthen Jack's faith in unity and support for one another support.

Jack faces physical challenges that push his endurance. A perilous mountain pass injures him and puts him in a vulnerable position. Lacking resources, he must depend on his ingenuity and the generosity of others to stay alive. This ordeal further humbles him and enhances his gratitude for life.

As Jack navigates these challenges, he views them as essential milestones in his transformation. Although painful, each trial molds him into a more empathetic and resilient person. These hardships create room within him for deeper wisdom and understanding strength.

During these moments, Jack came to a deep realization: true sovereignty involves confronting pain and hardship with courage and integrity rather than avoiding them. This insight would later become foundational in his teachings.

CHAPTER FOUR

The Sanctuary

JACK STANDS IN A vibrant valley, where time appears to pause, and nature's harmony is tangible. Captivated by the serene beauty around him, he imagines building a sanctuary for learning and personal growth. Within this refuge, those seeking wisdom can come together to reconnect with themselves and the environment.

Jack starts collecting materials from the valley, assisted by local villagers. His dream motivates those he encounters, and they contribute their skills to help realize the Sanctuary. Each structure they construct is filled with purpose, aiming to complement the land instead of overpowering it. Jack envisions a place where nature and humanity thrive together and harmoniously respect.

The Sanctuary serves as a guiding light for travelers and seekers from diverse backgrounds. Artists, healers, and thinkers bring their unique gifts, forming a vibrant mosaic of cultures and viewpoints. Jack organizes workshops focused on mindfulness, storytelling, and holistic wellness, informed by his experiences and ancient teachings tree.

One day, Jack discovers a child wandering alone in the valley. The child's innocence and sense of wonder evoke memories of his own youth, leading to a pivotal realization: the Sanctuary should also care for the younger generation. He starts creating programs for children, educating them on the values of self-awareness, compassion, and connection to Earth steward-ship.

Jack's evenings in the valley transform into moments of tranquil contemplation. Under the starlit sky, he reflects on his personal journey and the mission of the Sanctuary. Each night, the mur-murs of the ancient tree resonate through the rustling leaves, validating his direction and inspiring him to dream further.

The Sanctuary's Garden serves as its heart – a place for healing and sustenance. Jack, alongside the community, cultivates rare herbs and medicinal plants, sharing their benefits with those in need. Tending to the soil becomes a metaphor for growth and connection, strengthening the Sanctuary's role mission.

As the Sanctuary flourishes, Jack delights in observing the changes in its guests. Visitors come weighed down by fears yet depart with fresh clarity and a sense of purpose. The Sanctuary evolves from a mere physical location into a beacon of hope and renewal.

Jack begins chronicling his journey and the experiences of the Sanctuary's visitors. His accounts motivate others and extend the Sanctuary's message well beyond its immediate reach valley.

One evening, as a golden sunset cast a warm glow over the Sanctuary, Jack recognizes it as a living embodiment of all he has learned. It serves not just as a refuge but as a bridge – a space where past lessons intersect with his future aspirations.

CHAPTER FIVE

Workshop Retreats

Mindfulness Workshops

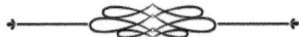

In the peaceful environment of the sanctuary, mindfulness work-shops aimed to nurture a strong sense of presence and awareness. Participants took part in guided practices, learning to notice their thoughts and emotions without judgment. By walking mindfully through serene gardens or engaging in silent reflection by a calm pond, they explored the beauty of being present. Mindfulness emerged as a means to cultivate inner peace, alleviate stress, and forge a deeper connection with the energy of the earth.

Meditation Retreats

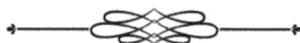

The meditation retreats offered a refuge within a refuge. Participants engaged in guided meditation sessions, exploring different techniques to calm their minds and access inner wisdom. Some chose to meditate in the enchanting chambers decorated with natural elements, while others found peace beneath the ancient trees. These retreats went beyond relaxation; they created a setting for individuals to explore their consciousness, uncovering hidden potentials and tapping into the universal energy that permeated the sanctuary.

Holistic Well-being Programs

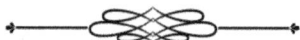

The holistic well-being programs acknowledged the connection between the mind, body, and spirit. Workshops highlighted holistic nutrition, herbal remedies from gardens, and methods that combined physical and spiritual health. Participants learned about the healing benefits of garden plants, making herbal teas and salves with guidance from experienced practitioners. Outdoor yoga and movement classes prompted participants to synchronize their breath with nature's rhythm, fostering a sense of bond with both nature and their own bodies.

Nature Immersion Retreats

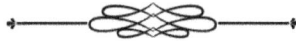

In addition to traditional workshops, the sanctuary hosted nature immersion retreats that led participants into the depths of the surrounding wilderness. Under the guidance of experienced naturalists and wisdom keepers, these retreats fostered a deep connection with the earth through sensory experiences. Engaging in activities like forest bathing and starlit night walks, participants explored the therapeutic advantages of nature, grounding themselves in its innate wisdom.

Community Circles and Wisdom Sharing

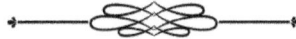

The workshops went beyond the structured sessions and developed into informal community gatherings. Participants exchanged their experiences, insights, and challenges in these circles. Elders and healers from different traditions were invited to share their wisdom, creating a rich tapestry of diverse viewpoints. These gatherings were essential in establishing a supportive community, celebrating the collective journey towards sovereignty while valuing each person's wisdom.

Empowering Children with Self-Awareness, Compassion, and Stewardship

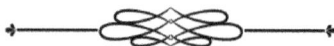

This workshop is designed to guide children through a journey of self-discovery, empathy, and environmental stewardship. Over five days, participants will explore themes of self-awareness, compassion, and connection to nature through creative activities, mindfulness practices, and hands-on experiences. The program fosters a sense of empowerment and responsibility, encouraging children to make thoughtful decisions and contribute to the well-being of their communities and the planet.

Children will engage in activities such as crafting personal totems, participating in group discussions on empathy, and creating eco-friendly art projects. They will also connect with nature by planting seeds, learning about ecosystems, and taking a pledge to protect the Earth. The final day celebrates their journey with a vision board exercise and a closing ceremony, leaving them inspired to carry forward the values of sovereignty and stewardship.

Essentially, the workshops at the Sanctuary of Sovereignty transcended traditional educational programs; they were immersive experiences encouraging participants to delve into their inner selves, connect with the natural world's energies, and nurture a harmonious relationship with themselves and the wider community. The sanctuary served as a dynamic classroom, where foundations of mindfulness, meditation, and holistic well-being were built to facilitate profound transformations within every individual.

Chapter Six

Call to Expansion

AFTER ESTABLISHING THE SANCTUARY as a site of transformation, Jack starts receiving requests from far-off regions to share his teachings. Initially, he is reluctant, doubting whether he can capture the Sanctuary's spirit in new environments. However, he recognizes that the tenets of sovereignty and resilience are universal and able to flourish anywhere. Motivated by a strong sense of purpose, he sets out on a journey that extends well beyond the valley, bringing the Sanctuary's essence to a broader audience world.

Jack's initial undertaking takes him to a coastal city where a dedicated group of activists strives to cultivate an urban oasis among towering skyscrapers. Their unwavering determination and ingenuity remind Jack of his own early challenges. Working together, they convert a vacant lot into a vibrant community garden and educational space. The endeavor faces several obstacles – opposition from city officials, limited resources, and skepticism from residents – but Jack's expertise and support enable the group to persevere.

The garden emerges as a symbol of hope in the city, demonstrating that even in highly urbanized areas, nature and community can flourish.

From the city, Jack journeys to a remote desert community grappling with severe drought and ecological decline. There, he encounters a group of indigenous leaders who have traditionally cared for the land. They educate Jack on their time-honored practices that prioritize harmony and acknowledge natural cycles. In response, Jack introduces methods for rainwater harvesting and sustainable farming. This exchange proves enriching for both sides, as Jack discovers that the Sanctuary's principles are not novel but rather grounded in ancient wisdom that has been overlooked by many. Together, they develop a resilience model that rejuvenates the land and fortifies the community.

Jack's journey continues to a bustling trade hub where cultural diversity is both a strength and a source of tension. Here, he facilitates workshops that bring together people from different backgrounds to share their stories and skills. Through dialogue and collaboration, barriers begin to dissolve, and a sense of unity emerges. Jack sees firsthand how the Sanctuary's empathy and mutual support ethos can bridge divides, fostering connections that transcend differences.

As Jack's work gains momentum, he is invited to speak at international gatherings and forums. While these opportunities amplify his message, they also test his ability to stay true to the Sanctuary's roots. Jack wrestles with the challenge of scaling an idea without diluting its essence. He often returns to the original Sanctuary in the valley to ground himself, seeking clarity under the ancient tree that first inspired his journey.

Jack has created a network of Sanctuaries, each distinct but connected by a common vision. He discovers that the movement's true power resides not in its growth but in how deeply it affects individuals and communities. The Sanctuaries serve as catalysts for change, demonstrating that sovereignty is a collective journey that flourishes through connections and shared goals.

CHAPTER SEVEN

Unity Amidst Diversity

As JACK TRAVELS THROUGH different cultures and traditions, he feels humbled by the rich diversity of human experiences. Each encounter teaches him something new as he observes how various societies uniquely convey universal truths. In one village, he discovers the significance of storytelling as an oral tradition that safeguards history and wisdom. In another, he finds that music can cross linguistic boundaries and evoke shared emotions, fostering connections that transcend cultural differences.

Jack recognizes that true unity celebrates differences instead of erasing them while also identifying common values. His collaboration with artists, educators, and healers worldwide emphasizes humanity's pursuit of connection and meaning. At a remote artist retreat, he observes how creativity has the power to heal emotional wounds. He engages in artistic creation with others who articulate their struggles and triumphs in their artwork. This journey reveals to Jack that art bridges the gap between individuals who might otherwise feel isolated by distance distances.

In a vibrant city, Jack collaborates with educators committed to empowering the youth. They create programs that merge traditional wisdom with modern practices, highlighting the importance of empathy and teamwork. Jack's concepts on mindfulness and interconnectedness strongly resonate with educators who envision a more harmonious future education.

Jack also spends time with healers who draw upon ancient practices to restore community balance. These individuals teach him how to merge physical, emotional, and spiritual healing into a cohesive whole. Through their guidance, Jack learns the significance of ritual and the deep respect many cultures have for their natural environment.

The diversity Jack encounters challenges him to re-evaluate his beliefs and adapt his teachings. He finds that resilience, creativity, and empathy are universal values, but how they are expressed varies profoundly. This realization enriches his understanding of sovereignty as a dynamic concept that evolves by blending perspectives.

Jack begins to see himself not as a teacher but as a facilitator of dialogue and exchange. He recognizes that each community he visits offers him as much wisdom as he brings to them. This humility deepens his connections and allows his message to flourish in ways he never imagined.

Jack has forged a network of collaborators who inspire one another to continue their work. The bonds he forms testify that unity does not require uniformity but rather a shared commitment to growth and understanding.

CHAPTER EIGHT

Shadows Within

JACK INCREASINGLY FEELS THE weight of leadership. The immense responsibility of steering a global movement often makes him feel isolated as if the Sanctuary's success has pulled him away from his initial purpose. Nights that used to be filled with quiet contemplation under starry skies now turn into sleepless stretches of doubt, leading Jack to question if he truly embodies the lessons, he teaches others.

Jack's internal struggle becomes increasingly evident to those closest to him. His once-unshakable confidence seems to waver, and his interactions grow strained as he grapples with feelings of inadequacy. The Sanctuary, now a thriving network of communities, requires constant attention. Jack feels the burden of every decision, fearing that a single misstep could unravel years of effort.

In his turmoil, Jack receives a letter from an old friend who was one of the Sanctuary's earliest visitors. The letter recounts the profound impact the Sanctuary had on their life, reminding Jack of the power of his work. This message becomes a turning point, igniting a desire to reconnect with the very roots of his journey.

Jack retreats from the demands of leadership and retreats to the original Sanctuary in the valley. He spends days walking among the gardens and meditating under the ancient tree. Slowly, the familiar whispers return, reminding him that sovereignty begins within. The tree's presence rekindles his sense of purpose, teaching him that leadership does not mean carrying every burden alone.

During his retreat, Jack is visited by members of the Sanctuary community, who share stories of their struggles and triumphs. Their words help him realize that his role is not to provide all the answers but to empower others to find their paths. The strength of the Sanctuary lies in its collective spirit, not in Jack himself alone.

Jack's time in solitude enables him to confront the fears and insecurities he had buried beneath layers of responsibility. He journals extensively, revealing patterns of self-doubt and perfectionism that had obscured his vision. By facing these shadows, Jack begins to heal, emerging with a renewed sense of awareness and clarity.

When Jack returns to his role, he approaches leadership with newfound humility and openness. He delegates responsibilities more freely, trusting the capable hands of his nurtured community. This shift lightens his burden and strengthens the Sanctuary, allowing it to evolve beyond his vision.

Jack stands again under the ancient tree, symbolizing his enduring journey. The whispers now carry a message of reassurance: that sovereignty is a continuous process, a balance of strength and vulnerability, and that even the most potent leaders must occasionally seek solace and renewal.

CHAPTER NINE

Legacy of the Sanctuary

As Jack stood under the ancient tree, he contemplated the journey that had led him back to this point. Initially a solitary vision in a peaceful valley, the Sanctuary transformed into a vibrant network of communities around the world. Each Sanctuary possessed its own distinct character, influenced by the local culture, environment, and the needs of its caretakers. Despite their differences, all were united by a common belief – a dedication to sovereignty, harmony, and resilience.

The original Sanctuary remained the heart of this movement, its gardens and meeting spaces now bustling with activity. Visitors from distant lands came to witness the birthplace of an idea that had transformed lives. Artists painted vivid murals depicting the Sanctuary's journey, while storytellers recounted Jack's odyssey to inspire the next generation. These narratives served as both a tribute and a call to action, reminding all who visited that sovereignty was a journey without an end.

Jack strolled through the grounds, noticing how the Sanctuary had expanded beyond his original vision. He witnessed children engaging in permaculture education in the gardens, their laughter blending with the buzz of bees. He observed elders sharing tales around a fire, connecting generations with wisdom and warmth. The Sanctuary had evolved into more than just a location; it was a vibrant, living representation of its ideals championed.

One day, Jack met a young leader who had just started a Sanctuary in a busy city. She discussed the difficulties she encountered in applying the philosophy to an urban setting, where space was limited and the community sometimes seemed disconnected. Nevertheless, she had effectively established rooftop gardens, communal areas, and initiatives that brought neighbors together. Her perseverance reminded Jack of his own early challenges and instilled a sense of pride in him. The seeds he had sown had flourished in unexpected places.

While listening to the leaders from other Sanctuaries, Jack understood that the movement thrived on its diversity. Each community had uniquely interpreted the core principles, weaving together various approaches that enhanced the entire group. Some Sanctuaries prioritized ecological restoration, whereas others highlighted education, art, or healing. Collectively, they created a mosaic of human potential, demonstrating that sovereignty could truly flourish anywhere.

The ancient tree Jack stood beneath had observed his entire journey. Its branches reached towards the sky, symbolizing growth, and resilience. Jack frequently listened to its whispers, discovering comfort and direction in its stillness. On this evening, as the sun sank below the horizon, he experienced a deep sense of tranquility. The project he had started was no longer solely his; it now belonged to everyone who had joined him.

During his later years, Jack dedicated himself to recording his teachings. He wrote extensively about both the obstacles and successes encountered while establishing the Sanctuary movement, intending to offer guidance for future advocates. His writings highlighted the significance of humility, adaptability, and trust within a team. Jack believed that true leaders are those who empower others to take the initiative lead.

As Jack looked up at the stars, he felt immense gratitude for those who had journeyed with him, the communities that had supported his vision, and a world open to change. He understood that the Sanctuary's real legacy would not lie in its physical structures but in the lives it had impacted and the hope it had nurtured. After all, sovereignty is a journey, not a final goal, and it will persist long after he is gone.

CHAPTER TEN

Finding Your True Purpose

A Guide to Rediscovering Direction When You Feel Lost

UNCOVERING YOUR PURPOSE ISN'T a universal experience. It's a deeply personal path that often involves stripping away societal conditioning and self-doubt to find your true self. This book provides a clear and practical method for assisting you in this journey, beginning with gaining insight into your identity beneath the surface.

Step 1: Reflect on Your Passions and Interests

One of the first steps in uncovering your purpose is identifying the activities, topics, or experiences that spark your enthusiasm. Ask yourself:

- *What activities cause you to lose track of time? Recall moments when you've been so absorbed in something that hours seemed like minutes. This "flow state" often indicates your passions.*

- *What hobbies or interests have you consistently enjoyed throughout the years? These may provide insight into what genuinely fulfills you.*

This section includes reflective journaling prompts to help you dig deeper. For example, you might list ten activities that bring you joy and identify emerging patterns.

Step 2: Identify Your Core Values

Your purpose connects deeply with your core values. This book assists you in identifying those values through various exercises like:

- Writing down what you admire most in others, these qualities often reflect your values.

- Reflect on decisions you've made that felt deeply satisfying and analyze what values those decisions aligned with.

You'll craft a "Values Map" that serves as a compass, helping you stay true to what matters most as you explore your purpose.

Step 3: Understand the Impact You Want to Make

Purpose often entails contributing to something greater than one-self. To discover this, ask:

- *What global issues are you most passionate about solving?*

- *What type of legacy do you wish to leave behind?*

This section provides practical tools, such as a "Legacy Work-sheet," to help you imagine your ideal future and impact. This will enable you to connect with your larger sense of meaning.

Step 4: Analyze Patterns in Your Past and Present

Your life story holds valuable clues about your purpose. You can uncover insights about your unique path by examining recurring themes, challenges you've overcome, and experiences that have shaped you.

- *Reflect on moments when you felt most alive and fulfilled.* What were you doing, and why did it matter to you?

- *Consider the struggles you've faced and the strengths you developed because of them.* These strengths can become the foundation for your purpose.

Step 5: Learn from Real-Life Examples

Sometimes, seeing how others have navigated their journeys is the best way to find clarity. The book shares inspiring stories of individuals who felt lost but discovered their purpose by aligning with their authentic desires. For instance:

- A corporate executive who pivoted to a career in environmental advocacy after realizing her passion for nature conservation.

- A teacher who started a nonprofit for underserved youth turned his struggles into a mission to help others.

These examples illustrate that, no matter where you are, you can create a meaningful life that aligns with your values and passions.

Step 6: Craft Your Purpose Statement

Once you've explored your passions, values, and desired impact, the book guides you through creating a purpose statement—an explicit, concise declaration of what drives you.

- Your purpose statement will answer: *"Who am I? What do I stand for? How do I want to contribute to the world?"*

- For example, "I am a storyteller who inspires others to embrace their creativity and live authentically."

This statement acts as your north star, providing direction and clarity as you navigate decisions and challenges in your life.

Step 7: Take Action to Live Your Purpose

Uncovering your purpose is only the beginning; the next step is to live it. The book includes actionable tips for integrating your purpose into your daily life, such as:

- Setting goals that align with your purpose.

- Building a support system of like-minded individuals.

- Regularly revisit and refine your purpose statement as you grow.

This comprehensive framework will give you the clarity and confidence to uncover your true purpose, even if you feel completely lost. This journey isn't about finding a pre-determined path; it's about creating one that feels authentically *yours*.

CHAPTER ELEVEN

The Transformative Power of Mindset Shifts

OVERCOMING FEAR AND SELF-DOUBT TO UNLOCK YOUR POTENTIAL

FEAR AND SELF-DOUBT AFFECT everyone, but they don't need to dictate your life. This book delves into how changing your mindset can turn these feelings into opportunities for growth instead of overwhelming obstacles. By providing actionable strategies and valuable insights, you will discover how to change your perception and reaction to fear and self-doubt, empowering you to advance confidently and clearly.

Understanding the Role of Fear and Self-Doubt

Fear and self-doubt often indicate that you are venturing into the unknown – an essential aspect of growth and transformation. Rather than viewing them as hurdles, this book encourages you to see them as natural and even necessary signs that you are pushing beyond your comfort zone. You will explore:

- Why fear often stems from uncertainty rather than actual danger.

- How self-doubt is rooted in societal conditioning and past experiences.

- The neuroscience behind fear responses and how to rewire your brain to manage them effectively.

Mindset Shift 1: Seeing Fear as a Sign of Growth

Fear is often misinterpreted as a signal to halt, yet it can serve as a powerful guide. This book shows you how to:

- Identify when fear is protecting you versus when it's holding you back.

- Reframe fear as a sign that you're stepping into new opportunities for growth.

- Use visualization techniques to reduce fear's intensity and replace it with excitement.

For example, instead of thinking, *"I'm scared, so I shouldn't do this,"* you'll learn to say, *"I'm scared because this is new and meaningful, which means it's worth pursuing."*

Mindset Shift 2: Reframing Failure as Feedback

Failure isn't the end—it's a valuable teacher. This book provides tools to help you:

- Break free from the "all-or-nothing" thinking that makes failure feel catastrophic.

- View each setback as an opportunity to learn and adjust your approach.

- Develop a "growth mindset," where challenges are seen as improvement opportunities rather than proof of inadequacy.

Through relatable examples, such as inventors and entrepreneurs who turned failure into motivation for their success, you'll see how shifting your perspective can transform failures into stepping stones.

Mindset Shift 3: Challenging Limiting Beliefs

Limiting beliefs are the internal scripts that tell you, *"I'm not good enough," "I'll never succeed,"* or *"It's too late for me."* These beliefs often stem from past experiences or external judgments, but they don't have to define you. This book equips you to:

- Identify the limiting beliefs that are holding you back.

- Write counterarguments to these beliefs, using logic and evidence to disprove them.

- Replace negative self-talk with empowering affirmations.

For instance, instead of saying, *"I don't have what it takes,"* you'll learn to say, *"I have the skills and determination to figure this out."*

Actionable Exercises for Mindset Shifts

To help you internalize these mindset shifts, the book includes practical exercises such as:

1. **Counterargument Journaling**: Write your fears and doubts, then create rational, evidence-based rebuttals. For example, if your inner critic says, *"You'll never succeed,"* counter it with, *"I've succeeded in the past when I tried new things, and I'll succeed again."*

2. **Daily Affirmations**: Develop a habit of repeating posi-

tive affirmations each morning, such as *"I am capable of overcoming challenges"* or *"Fear is a sign that I'm growing."*

3. **Fear-Tracking Logs**: Keep a journal where you record moments of fear, what triggered them, and how you responded. Over time, you'll notice patterns and build a toolkit for managing fear effectively.

4. **Visualization Techniques**: Spend a few minutes each day imagining yourself succeeding at something that scares you. Visualization primes your brain for confidence and success.

Real-Life Stories of Transformation

The book shares inspiring stories of individuals who overcame fear and self-doubt by embracing these mindset shifts. For example:

- A young professional who went from fearing public speaking to delivering TED Talks by reframing her fear as excitement.

- A mother who returned to school after years of self-doubt, realizing it was never "too late" to pursue her dreams.

These examples illustrate how mindset shifts can lead to profound personal and professional transformations.

The Long-Term Benefits of Mindset Shifts

Adopting these new ways of thinking won't just help you conquer immediate challenges; they'll set the foundation for a lifetime of resilience and growth. Over time, you'll find that:

- Fear becomes less paralyzing and more manageable.

- Self-doubt is replaced with self-compassion and confidence.

- You approach challenges with curiosity and determination rather than avoidance.

By understanding and implementing these mindset shifts, you'll gain the tools to conquer fear and self-doubt, unlock your full potential, and lead a more confident, fulfilling life. This isn't just about thinking differently – it's about transforming how you live.

CHAPTER TWELVE

Crafting Your Personal Roadmap

A STEP-BY-STEP GUIDE TO ALIGNING YOUR LIFE WITH YOUR DREAMS

DREAMS ARE THE SEEDS of a fulfilling life, but without a clear plan, they often remain just that – dreams. This book provides a comprehensive, step-by-step process to turn your aspirations into actionable goals through a personalized roadmap. By following this framework, you'll clarify your vision and stay motivated and on track, even when life throws challenge your way.

Step 1: Vision Mapping

The first step in creating your roadmap is to define your ideal future with clarity and intention. Vision mapping helps you articulate what you truly want and why it matters. Here's how:

- **Create a Vision Board**: Gather images, quotes, and symbols representing your dreams and arrange them on a physical or digital board. This visual representation keeps your goals front and center in your mind.

- **Write a Vision Narrative**: Describe your ideal life as if it's already happening. Be specific: Where are you? What are you doing? Who are you with? How does it feel? Writing this narrative activates your imagination and helps solidify your goals.

- **Reflect on Key Life Areas**: Consider career, relationships, health, personal growth, and leisure. What does success look like in each of these?

This step ensures a vivid picture of your future, providing the foundation for the roadmap.

Step 2: Goal Setting

Big dreams can feel overwhelming until you break them down into manageable pieces. The SMART goal framework helps ensure your goals are Specific, Measurable, Achievable, Relevant, and Time-bound:

- **Break Down Big Dreams**: Start with your long-term vision (5–10 years) and break it into smaller milestones for 1 year, 6 months, and 3 months. For example, if your dream is to start a business, a 6-month milestone might be developing a business plan.

- **Prioritize Goals**: Identify which goals matter most and will have the most significant impact. Focus on these first to avoid feeling overwhelmed.

- **Set Micro-Goals**: Define weekly or daily tasks contributing to your larger goals. For example, "Write 500 words daily" for an aspiring author.

By structuring your goals this way, you'll create a clear path from your current position to your desired position.

Step 3: Daily Planning

Integrate your goals into your daily life to turn your roadmap into action. This step is about bridging the gap between dreams and consistent progress:

- **Time-Blocking**: Schedule dedicated blocks for specific tasks related to your goals. For example, set aside 30 minutes each morning to work on personal development or fitness.

- **Priority Setting**: Use tools like the Eisenhower Matrix to categorize tasks as urgent, essential, or non-essential. Focus on what truly moves the needle.

- **Morning and Evening Routines**: Incorporate your

roadmap into your daily rituals. Start your day by reviewing your goals and planning tasks, and end by reflecting on your progress.

Daily planning ensures that your roadmap doesn't stay theoretical – it becomes part of your everyday life.

Step 4: Progress Tracking

Tracking your progress helps you stay motivated and identify areas for improvement. This book offers simple yet effective tools to measure your achievements:

- **Goal Trackers**: Use habit trackers, apps, or spreadsheets to monitor daily and weekly tasks. Seeing progress visually can be incredibly motivating.

- **Review Milestones Regularly**: Set aside time each month to evaluate your progress toward your milestones. Are you on track? What's working well? What needs adjustment?

- **Celebrate Wins**: Recognize and reward yourself for hitting milestones, no matter how small. Celebrations reinforce positive behavior and keep you engaged.

- **Adjust for Flexibility**: Life is unpredictable, so be willing to adapt your roadmap. If something isn't working, pivot rather than abandoning your goals entirely.

You'll stay focused and maintain momentum by tracking progress, even when faced with challenges.

Step 5: Adapting to Life's Twists and Turns

A successful roadmap isn't rigid; it's dynamic and responsive. This book teaches you how to:

- **Expect Challenges**: Understand that setbacks are part of the journey. Have contingency plans in place for when things don't go as expected.

- **Reassess Your Vision**: Periodically revisit your vision to ensure it aligns with your evolving priorities and desires.

- **Stay Resilient**: Use the mindset shifts discussed earlier to navigate obstacles with confidence and optimism.

Flexibility ensures that your roadmap remains relevant and realistic, no matter how life evolves.

The Roadmap to Your Dreams

This step-by-step guide combines vision mapping, goal setting, daily planning, and progress tracking to help you transform vague aspirations into tangible achievements. You'll gain clarity, stay motivated, and maintain direction, even when uncertain. Most importantly, this roadmap empowers you to align your actions with your dreams, creating a life that feels purposeful and fulfilling daily.

CHAPTER THIRTEEN

Simple Daily Practices for Growth

CULTIVATING CONFIDENCE, RESILIENCE, AND INNER PEACE EVERY DAY

SIGNIFICANT CHANGES DON'T HAPPEN overnight they result from consistent, intentional habits that shape your mindset and emotional well-being over time. This book introduces simple daily practices designed to help you cultivate confidence, resilience, and inner peace. These practices require a few minutes each day but can create profound shifts in how you think, feel, and act.

Morning Affirmations: Start Your Day with Empowering Statements

Your first thoughts in the morning set the tone for the rest of your day. Morning affirmations are a powerful way to replace negative or limiting thoughts with empowering, positive ones.

- **Why Affirmations Work**: They help rewire your brain by creating new neural pathways that support self-belief and confidence.

- **How to Practice**: Choose 3–5 affirmations that resonate with your goals and values. For example:

  - *"I am capable of achieving great things."*

  - *"I face challenges with confidence and grace."*

  - *"I deserve happiness and success."*
    Say these affirmations out loud or write them down each morning to reinforce a positive mindset.

Over time, these affirmations will become internalized, shaping your thoughts and actions throughout the day.

Gratitude Journaling: Shift Your Focus to Abundance

Gratitude is one of the simplest yet most powerful ways to cultivate inner peace and resilience. Focusing on what you have rather than your lack naturally reduces stress and increases happiness.

- **Why Gratitude Journaling Works**: It trains your brain to notice and appreciate the positive aspects of your life, even during challenging times.

- **How to Practice**: Spend five minutes each morning or evening writing down 3–5 things you're grateful for. Be specific:

  - Instead of "I'm grateful for my family," try "I'm grateful for the kind words my partner said to me today."

  - Instead of "I'm grateful for my job," try "I'm grateful for the opportunity to lead a successful presentation at work."

This simple practice helps you develop an abundance and appreciation mindset, fostering confidence and emotional resilience.

Mindfulness Exercises: Center Yourself with Breathing and Meditation

Mindfulness is the practice of staying present in the moment, which can help you navigate stress and challenges with greater clarity and calm.

- **Why Mindfulness Works**: It reduces anxiety, improves focus, and enhances your ability to respond rather than react to situations.

- **How to Practice**:

  - **Breathing Techniques**: Spend 2–5 minutes focusing on your breath. Try the 4-7-8 technique: inhale for four counts, hold for seven, and exhale for eight counts. This activates your parasympathetic nervous system, reducing stress.

  - **Mini Meditations**: You can use guided meditations or sit quietly, focusing on a single point, such as your breath or a soothing word (e.g., "peace").

  - **Body Scans**: Spend a few moments focusing on different parts of your body and releasing tension as you go.

These exercises help you cultivate a sense of calm and control, making it easier to face daily challenges confidently.

Visualization: Reinforce Belief in Your Potential

Visualization is a powerful technique for building confidence by mentally rehearsing success. It primes your brain to recognize opportunities and act decisively when they arise.

- **Why Visualization Works**: Studies show that mental rehearsal activates the same neural pathways as physical practice, boosting performance and self-belief.

- **How to Practice**:

  - Spend 5 minutes imagining yourself succeeding at a specific goal. For example, if you're preparing for a presentation, visualize yourself speaking confidently, engaging the audience, and receiving positive feedback.

  - To achieve your goal, include as many senses as possible. Imagine how it feels, looks, and sounds.

  - Pair visualization with an empowering mantra, like *"I've got this."*

This daily practice helps you build a strong mental image of your potential, reinforcing the belief that you can achieve your dreams.

Why These Practices Work Together

When practiced regularly, these simple habits have a compounding effect:

- **Confidence**: Morning affirmations and visualization build self-belief, creating a foundation of confidence that grows stronger each day.

- **Resilience**: Gratitude journaling and mindfulness exercises help you manage stress, stay grounded, and bounce back from setbacks more quickly.

- **Inner Peace**: The combined effect of gratitude, mindfulness, and visualization fosters a sense of calm and contentment, allowing you to navigate life with clarity and ease.

Making It a Routine

To make these practices a consistent part of your life:

- Start small—choose one practice, then gradually add others.

- Pair practices with existing habits (e.g., gratitude journaling with your morning coffee).

- Stay on track with prompts or reminders, such as sticky notes, apps, or alarms.

Dedicating 10–15 minutes daily to these practices will build confidence, resilience, and inner peace, which will support your goals and help you live a more fulfilling life.

CHAPTER FOURTEEN

Turning Failures Into Fuel

TRANSFORMING PAST SETBACKS INTO STEPPING STONES FOR GROWTH

FAILURE IS OFTEN VIEWED as an endpoint, a source of shame or regret. However, it can also catalyze growth and transformation when approached with the right mindset. This section explores practical strategies for releasing the emotional weight of past failures, gaining valuable insights, and using those experiences as stepping stones toward success.

Practice Self-Compassion: Forgive Yourself and Embrace Kindness

Self-compassion is the foundation for moving past failure. Often, we are our harshest critics, replaying mistakes in our minds and berating ourselves for not living up to expectations. Learning to treat yourself with kindness can break this cycle.

- **Why It Matters**: Studies show that self-compassion reduces anxiety and fosters resilience, making it easier to bounce back from setbacks.

- **How to Practice Self-Compassion**:

  - **Acknowledge Your Humanity**: Remind yourself that everyone makes mistakes and experiences failure. It's a natural part of growth.

  - **Change Your Inner Dialogue**: When self-critical thoughts arise, reframe them with supportive statements. For example, replace *"I'm such a failure"* with *"I'm learning and growing from this experience."*

  - **Engage in Self-Care**: Treat yourself like a close friend going through a tough time offer encouragement, rest, and patience.

This practice helps you build a healthier relationship with yourself, freeing you from the cycle of self-blame and shame.

Reframe Failure: Turn Regrets into Lessons and Wisdom

Failure becomes meaningful when you can extract lessons from the experience. Instead of focusing on what went wrong, shift your perspective to identify what you gained.

- **Why It Matters**: Reframing failure allows you to see it as a temporary setback rather than a permanent reflection of your abilities.

- **How to Reframe Failure**:

  - **Ask Reflective Questions**:

    - What did I learn about myself, others, or the situation?

    - What would I do differently next time?

    - How did this failure shape me for the better?

  - **Focus on Growth**: Recognize that every failure builds skills, resilience, or clarity that you didn't have before. For example, a failed job interview might teach you to better prepare for future opportunities.

  - **Keep a "Failure Journal"**: Document your failures and lessons learned. Over time, you'll see how setbacks have contributed to your progress.

Reframing helps you shift from dwelling on mistakes to viewing them as valuable learning experiences.

Create Symbolic Closure: Let Go of Regret with Rituals

Sometimes, past failures feel like an emotional weight you can't shake. A symbolic act of closure can help you release that burden and move forward.

- **Why It Matters**: Symbolic closure provides a sense of finality and allows you to process lingering emotions healthily.

- **How to Create Closure**:

  - **Write a Letter to Your Past Self**: Address your past self with empathy and understanding. Acknowledge the pain of the failure, but also highlight the growth and strength you've gained since then. Once written, you can keep the letter as a reminder or ceremonially destroy it to signify letting go.

  - **Create a Letting-Go Ritual**:

    - Write down the failure and associated emotions on a piece of paper.

- Burn, shred, or bury the paper as a symbolic act of releasing regret.

  ○ **Visualization Exercise**: Close your eyes and imagine the failure as a heavy object. Then, imagine yourself setting it down and walking away lighter and freer.

These rituals help you process emotions and create a psychological break from the past.

Build Resilience Through Failure

Resilience is the ability to recover quickly from setbacks. By embracing failure as an integral part of growth, you develop the emotional strength to face future challenges confidently.

- **Why It Matters**: Resilience helps you stay focused on long-term goals, even in adversity.

- **How to Build Resilience**:

  ○ **Develop a Growth Mindset**: Embrace the belief that your abilities and intelligence can be developed through effort and learning.

  ○ **Celebrate Small Wins**: Recognize and reward yourself for progress, no matter how small. This reinforces the idea that failure is a stepping stone to success.

  ○ **Surround Yourself with Support**: Share your experiences with trusted friends, mentors, or a support group. Hearing others' stories of overcoming failure can inspire and motivate you.

Resilience ensures that failure doesn't deter you but strengthens your resolve to keep moving forward.

Shift Your Relationship with Failure

To truly let go of past failures, you must redefine what failure means. Rather than seeing it as a negative outcome, view it as essential to growth and success.

- **Adopt the "Fail Forward" Mentality**: Accept that failure is inevitable in achieving your goals. Each failure brings you one step closer to success.

- **Redefine Success**: Success isn't the absence of failure it's the ability to learn, adapt, and persevere despite setbacks.

The Transformative Power of Letting Go

By practicing self-compassion, reframing failure, and engaging in symbolic closure, you can free yourself from the emotional weight of the past. These strategies help you move forward and enable you to use failure as a powerful tool for personal growth. Over time, you'll develop the confidence and resilience to face challenges head-on, turning every setback into a stepping stone on your journey to success.

CHAPTER FIFTEEN

Building Habits for Success

DAILY PRACTICES TO ACHIEVE YOUR GOALS WITH CONSISTENCY

HABITS SHAPE YOUR LIFE far more than occasional bursts of effort. They're the building blocks of success, helping you make steady progress toward your goals with less effort over time. This book delves into the science of habit formation and provides actionable strategies to build positive habits that stick.

The Science of Habits: Why They Matter

Habits are automated behaviors triggered by cues in your environment. Once formed, they require minimal willpower to maintain. Here's why they're crucial for achieving your goals:

- **Efficiency**: Habits allow you to perform essential tasks without overthinking, freeing up mental energy for creative or complex work.

- **Consistency**: Daily habits create minor, compounding improvements that yield significant long-term results.

- **Resilience**: Strong habits form a foundation, helping you stay grounded and focused even during challenging times.

This section introduces you to the habit loop a three-step process of *cue, routine, and reward*—and shows how to harness it for goal-setting.

Habit Stacking: Pair New Habits with Existing Ones

Habit stacking leverages the power of routines you already have to make it easier to build new ones. You create a natural sequence that reinforces both behaviors by anchoring a new habit to an established one.

- **Why It Works**: Adding a habit to an existing routine reduces the effort required to start. Your brain associates the two actions, making the new habit automatic.

- **How to Use Habit Stacking**:

  - Identify a daily habit you already have, such as brushing your teeth, brewing coffee, or checking your email.

  - Pair a new habit with the existing one. For example:

- After brushing your teeth, spend 2 minutes practicing gratitude.

- While waiting for your coffee to brew, do a quick stretching routine.

- Before checking your email, review your daily goals.

  ○ Write down your habit stack as a sentence: *"After [existing habit], I will [new habit]."*

This approach helps you incorporate new behaviors seamlessly into your routine.

Triggers and Rewards: The Keys to Habit Formation

Every habit begins with a trigger (or cue) that prompts the behavior and ends with a reward that reinforces it. Understanding these elements is essential for creating and maintaining habits.

- **Triggers**:

  ○ Use environmental cues. For example, Place a journal on your bedside table to remind you to write in it each morning.

  ○ Set time-based triggers: Start your workout at the same time every day.

- Create action-based triggers: Pair your new habit with an activity, like drinking water, every time you finish a meeting.

- **Rewards**:

  - Make the reward immediate and satisfying: Celebrate completing a habit with a positive affirmation or small treat.

  - Link habits to long-term rewards: Visualize how each habit contributes to your bigger goals. For example, consider daily exercise a step toward long-term health.

By carefully designing triggers and rewards, you make habits more appealing and easier to sustain.

Small Wins: Build Momentum with Manageable Habits

Significant changes often start with small, manageable actions. Focusing on tiny, achievable habits reduces overwhelm and builds momentum.

- **Why Small Wins Matter**: Small habits are easy to integrate into your routine and offer quick successes that motivate you to keep going.

- **How to Start with Small Wins**:

- ○ Break down big goals into micro-habits. For example:

  - Goal: Write a book.

  - Micro-habit: Write 50 words a day.

  - Goal: Get fit.

  - Micro-habit: Do five push-ups each morning.

- ○ Gradually increase the difficulty as the habit becomes ingrained. For example, writing 50 words daily might become 500, and doing five push-ups might lead to a complete workout.

- ○ Celebrate small successes to reinforce positive behavior.

These small wins create a ripple effect, making it easier to tackle more significant challenges over time.

Use a Habit Tracker to Stay Accountable

Tracking your habits helps you stay consistent and visually measure your progress. It also reinforces the habit loop by serving as a cue and a reward.

- **How to Use a Habit Tracker**:

  - ○ Choose a method that works for you, such as a paper

journal, mobile app, or spreadsheet.

- List the habits you want to track and mark off each day you complete them.

- Set a goal for streaks (e.g., completing a habit for 21 consecutive days) to motivate yourself.

- **Benefits of Habit Tracking**:

   - Provides a clear record of your efforts.

   - Identifies patterns, helping you see which habits stick and which need adjustment.

   - It offers a sense of accomplishment, especially when your streak grows.

The habit tracker template included in this book provides an easy-to-use format for monitoring your progress and celebrating wins.

Tips for Sustaining Long-Term Habits

Building habits is one thing; maintaining them is another. This book provides strategies to ensure your habits become part of your identity:

- **Focus on Identity, Not Outcomes**: Shift your mindset from *"I want to lose weight"* to *"I am someone who priori-*

tizes health."

- **Plan for Setbacks**: Accept that life happens and habits may falter. Have a plan to restart quickly without self-judgment.

- **Stack Rewards Over Time**: Tie habits to long-term rewards, like treating yourself to something special after completing a 30-day streak.

Cultivating habits is more than achieving individual goals it's about becoming the person you aspire to be. Mastering habit formation will create a foundation for lifelong growth and success. These daily practices, while small, lead to profound transformation when compounded over time. This book gives you the tools to build habits that bring you closer to your goals and shape a more confident, resilient, and fulfilled version of yourself.

CHAPTER SIXTEEN

Living Authentically on Your Terms

UNLOCKING THE SECRET TO AN UNAPOLOGETIC LIFE

LIVING AUTHENTICALLY MEANS ALIGNING with your true self, your values, desires, and unique identity, rather than conforming to societal expectations or external pressures. It's about embracing yourself and making choices that honor your truth. This section explores actionable strategies for cultivating authenticity, helping you live a life that feels profoundly fulfilling and unapologetically *yours*.

Tap Into Your Intuition: Trust Your Gut Instincts

Your intuition is your internal compass, guiding you toward decisions that align with your true self. However, modern life often drowns out this inner voice with external noise and societal expectations.

- **Why Intuition Matters**: Intuition is a reflection of your subconscious knowledge, shaped by your experiences, values, and emotions. It helps you make decisions that feel right even when logic alone can't provide clarity.

- **How to Tap Into Your Intuition**:

  - **Create Quiet Moments**: Spend time in silence or meditation to reconnect with your inner voice. This allows you to separate intuition from fear or doubt.

  - **Notice Physical Cues**: Pay attention to how your body reacts to decisions. A sense of ease or excitement often indicates alignment, while tension or discomfort may signal misalignment.

  - **Ask Reflective Questions**: When faced with a choice, ask yourself, *"Does this decision honor my values and bring me closer to the life I want?"*

  - **Trust the First Feeling**: Intuitive insights often appear quickly and feel instinctive. Trusting this initial reaction can guide you toward authenticity.

Tuning into your intuition helps you make choices that reflect who you truly are, even when they defy external expectations.

Set Boundaries: Honor Your Values and Priorities

Living authentically requires setting and maintaining boundaries to protect your time, energy, and emotional well-being. Boundaries empower you to say "no" to what doesn't serve you, creating space for what truly matters.

- **Why Boundaries Are Essential**: Without boundaries, you risk being pulled in directions that don't align with your values, leading to burnout, resentment, and a sense of disconnection from yourself.

- **How to Set Boundaries**:

  - **Identify Your Limits**: Reflect on situations where you feel drained, stressed, or unfulfilled. These are areas where boundaries are needed.

  - **Communicate Clearly**: Use assertive but respectful language to express your boundaries. For example: *"I'm unable to take on additional work this week, but I can revisit this next month."*

  - **Stick to Your Decisions**: Honor your boundaries consistently, even when it feels uncomfortable. This reinforces your commitment to yourself.

  - **Prioritize Your Values**: When deciding whether to say "yes" or "no," ask yourself if the request aligns with your priorities and long-term goals.

By setting boundaries, you protect your authentic self from being overshadowed by others' expectations or demands.

Embrace Vulnerability: Strengthen Your Connection to Yourself and Others

Vulnerability is often perceived as weakness, but it's actually a source of strength. Being open and honest about your struggles, emotions, and imperfections allows you to live authentically and fosters deeper connections with others.

- **Why Vulnerability Matters**: Vulnerability is the gateway to authenticity. It allows you to show up as your true self without fear of judgment, fostering trust and intimacy in relationships.

- **How to Embrace Vulnerability**:

  - **Acknowledge Your Feelings**: Instead of suppressing emotions, allow yourself to feel them fully and express them honestly.

  - **Share Your Story**: Open up about your experiences, even the difficult ones. Sharing your truth helps you release shame and builds empathy with others.

  - **Reframe Vulnerability as Courage**: Recognize that

showing your authentic self, even in the face of potential rejection, is an act of bravery.

- ○ **Practice Self-Compassion**: Treat yourself kindly when vulnerability feels uncomfortable or exposes insecurities.

By embracing vulnerability, you build the courage to live unapologetically and foster deeper, more authentic connections.

Let Go of Societal Expectations

Societal norms and external pressures can push you to live inauthentically, chasing goals that don't truly resonate with you. Breaking free from these expectations allows you to live life on your own terms.

- **Why It's Important**: Living for others' approval can lead to dissatisfaction and a lack of fulfillment. Authenticity requires defining success for yourself.

- **How to Release Societal Expectations**:

  - ○ **Challenge Norms**: Ask yourself if societal "rules" align with your values. For example, is climbing the corporate ladder your dream, or is it what you've been conditioned to pursue?

  - ○ **Redefine Success**: Create a personal definition of

success that reflects your passions, values, and desires.

- ○ **Surround Yourself with Support**: Seek out a community of like-minded individuals who celebrate your authenticity rather than pressuring you to conform.

Letting go of external expectations liberates you to create a life that feels uniquely yours.

Make Authenticity a Daily Practice

Authenticity isn't a one-time decision—it's a way of life. Small, consistent actions help you stay true to yourself every day.

- • **Daily Practices for Authentic Living**:

  - ○ **Start Each Day Intentionally**: Reflect on your values and how you can honor them in your daily choices.

  - ○ **Practice Honest Communication**: Speak your truth, even when it feels uncomfortable. Authenticity requires transparency.

  - ○ **Check in with Yourself**: At the end of each day, reflect on whether your actions aligned with your authentic self.

Authenticity becomes easier with practice, gradually reshaping your life to reflect your true self.

The Benefits of Living Authentically

When you live authentically and unapologetically, you unlock a life of:

- **Fulfillment**: Your actions and choices align with your values, leading to a deeper sense of purpose.

- **Confidence**: Trusting yourself and setting boundaries strengthens your self-worth.

- **Freedom**: Letting go of societal expectations allows you to live without fear of judgment.

- **Connection**: Vulnerability fosters stronger, more meaningful relationships.

Authenticity isn't just a goal; it's a journey of self-discovery and empowerment that leads to a life of greater joy, resilience, and personal fulfillment. Through the tools in this book, you'll develop the confidence and courage to live unapologetically on your terms.

CHAPTER SEVENTEEN

Empowering Affirmations

HARNESSING THE POWER OF WORDS TO EMBRACE YOUR TRUE SELF

USE THESE AFFIRMATIONS DAILY to align your mindset with confidence, resilience, and authenticity. Repeat them aloud, write them in your journal, or reflect on them during moments of quiet. These statements are designed to reinforce your belief in yourself and your ability to live unapologetically on your terms.

Affirmations for Confidence

- I am capable of achieving great things.

- I trust myself to make the right decisions for my life.

- I embrace challenges as opportunities to grow stronger.

- My unique qualities are my greatest strengths.

- I speak my truth with courage and clarity.

Affirmations for Resilience

- I can overcome any obstacle with grace and determination.

- Setbacks are stepping stones to my success.

- I learn and grow from every experience, good or bad.

- I release the past and focus on the opportunities of today.

- I have the power to bounce back stronger after every challenge.

Affirmations for Inner Peace

- I am at peace with who I am and where I am in my journey.

- I let go of fear and embrace the present moment.

- My mind is calm, my heart is open, and my soul is content.

- I am grateful for the abundance in my life.

- I create harmony in my life with ease and intention.

Affirmations for Authentic Living

- I honor my values and live in alignment with my true self.

- I give myself permission to say "no" to what doesn't serve me.

- I am free to live a life that reflects my unique purpose.

- I trust my intuition to guide me toward what feels right.

- I am unapologetically me, and that is enough.

Affirmations for Self-Love and Acceptance

- I love and accept myself exactly as I am.

- I deserve happiness, success, and love.

- I am worthy of the life I dream of.

- I am kind to myself and celebrate my progress, no matter how small.

- I embrace my imperfections as part of what makes me unique.

Affirmations for Goal Achievement

- I have the discipline and focus to achieve my goals.

- I am worthy of the success I am creating.

- I take consistent, inspired action toward my dreams.

- My efforts today are paving the way for my future success.

- I am unstoppable when I set my mind to something.

How to Use These Affirmations:

- Choose 3–5 affirmations that resonate with you each day.

- Repeat them in the morning to set a positive tone or in the evening to reflect on your progress.

- Write them in your journal or on sticky notes placed where you'll see them often (e.g., on your mirror or desk).

Affirmations are a daily reminder of your strength, potential, and ability to live a life that is authentic and fulfilling. Let them inspire and empower you to take meaningful steps toward your goals every day.

Conclusion

As the final chords of Jack's journey resonate, we are reminded of the infinite potential within each of us.

His odyssey is a testament to the power of courage, connection, and transformation.

Jack illuminated the path toward sovereignty through his trials and triumphs, inviting us all to awaken the harmony within.

Dear reader, may the essence of Jack's journey inspire you to embrace your sovereignty and navigate your path with resilience and grace.

Carry his legacy as a beacon of hope and may your journey weave a tapestry of harmony and enlightenment for generations to come.

About the Author

Sabrina Winterstone is an emerging writer with a passion for storytelling. Although new to the literary world, she has always been captivated by the power of words and the magic of bringing characters and ideas to life. With a deep curiosity for exploring different genres and themes, Sabrina is committed to honing their craft and continuing to write stories that resonate with readers. This is just the beginning of their journey, and they look forward to sharing more of their work as they grow as an author.

www.ingramcontent.com/pod-product-compliance
Lightning Source LLC
Chambersburg PA
CBHW051259020426
42333CB00026B/3275